Sharing the Road

A Journey through Parkinson's Disease

SHARING THE ROAD

A Journey through Parkinson's Disease

Case J. Boot

DORDT COLLEGE PRESS

Cover design and layout by Carla Goslinga

Copyright © 2011 by Case J. Boot

Printed in the United States of America.

Dordt College Press   www.dordt.edu/dordt_press
498 Fourth Avenue NE
Sioux Center, Iowa 51250
United States of America

ISBN 978-0-932914-89-7

Library of Congress Cataloging-in-Publication Data:
2011929114

DEDICATION

First of all, I would like to dedicate this book, *Sharing the Road, A Journey Through Parkinson's Disease*, to my wife Aly. She has worked numerous hours when I was a student, and she was a model for our whole family by working late hours and teaching knitting and other crafts to people in the community. Now, she works lovingly and tirelessly to help me in my journey with Parkinson's. It's her journey, too.

I would also like to dedicate this book to our four children: Tony, Tres, Deb, and Reggie. When they were young they shared lots of family travels and met guests from all over the world. Although now they live far away, as I travel this challenging road through Parkinson's disease, they support me with their love and encouragement.

On our 40th
wedding anniversary.

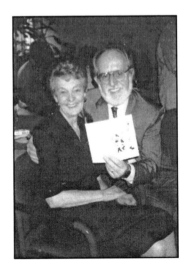

TABLE OF CONTENTS

PREFACE

I have the privilege of being Case Boot's pastor as he learns to live with Parkinson's disease. It is a disease that one must accommodate in one's life as there is no "cure." Yes, there are medications that help mask the symptoms, and there are activities that will help one deal with the effects of Parkinson's, but ultimately one has to share the road with Parkinson's disease. It can be a lonely journey as one may wonder if anyone else knows what he or she is experiencing. Case Boot, my former professor and now member of East Hill Community Christian Reformed Church where I serve, shares his journey in these pages as one who is learning to live with Parkinson's.

Although Case and I both had Rocky Mountain House as our home town, I was very young when the Boots left town so I first really met Case and Aly Boot when I attended Dordt College in Sioux Center, Iowa. Case was a professor of linguistics, and I had the opportunity to take a Dutch class from Professor Boot to fulfill a modern language requirement. I look back on those classes and realize I have forgotten much of the vocabulary and the grammar; I do not remember all the "het" words or the "de" words. But what I do remember is a professor who passionately loved Jesus and the worldview that Christ is Lord of all parts of life, with every square inch of creation needing to be brought back into relationship with Christ. I also remember an off-handed comment made by Professor Boot in one of the Dutch classes, that in his opinion we will be doing linguistics in heaven! That comment was the catalyst for my view about heaven and earth and redemption to be forever reformed.

It is important to me to reflect on my memories of Case because it is easy for us to observe someone with Parkinson's and let the Parkinson's shape our view of the person. It is important to remember this is a person who likes to laugh, love, talk, think, and cry. This is a person who ran and jumped and played, a person who is a husband, a father, a baker, a teacher, a professor, a coach, a mentor, and a friend.

When I moved to Vernon, BC in 2004, Case was serving the church as an elder. His speech and walk demonstrated that Parkinson's was shaping an increasingly larger part of his life. Case continued to remain positive however, walking his dog dutifully every day and serving in the church with joy.

I remember praying in church one Sunday for Case "as he struggles with Parkinson's disease." Case called me later and told me not to pray that way as he no longer "struggles" with Parkinson's. What I understood him to mean is that God had given him the grace to be able to journey with Parkinson's disease or as he says to share the road with it. The journey is not an easy stroll through a park but a hike through very difficult terrain. Parkinson's disease is a road hog and wants an increasingly bigger part of the road. But Case has learned, and is continuing to learn, to live with this disease. He is still a professor at heart, and willingly shares his story to teach us about the journey with Parkinson's disease.

Andrew Vander Leek

INTRODUCTION

Let me introduce myself so the story of my journey with Parkinson's disease has some context for you as a reader. I was born Kornelis Johannes Boot (Case) in 1932 in the Netherlands to a middle class family. I was the oldest son of a family of eleven children. My heritage was rooted in faith in Jesus Christ and, like my father before me, in the skills of a baker. In 1950 our family immigrated to Canada, first to the Lethbridge area of Alberta, and then to the Red Deer area. There I met my wife Aly. We married in 1955 and moved to Rocky Mountain House. I owned and operated Heatherdale Bakery there; we started our family (four children) and were active in the Christian Reformed Church (CRC). Then, God brought a new turn in the road.

The summer of 1961, an American CRC preacher was the main speaker at a Young People's Camp at Sylvan Lake. Soon the rumour spread throughout central Alberta that he was a preacher with a real Calvinist world-and-life-view, something dear to my heart. One summer evening, Aly and I attended an evening session, and we were gripped by the speaker's vision. The speaker was Rev. B. J. Haan, president of Dordt College in Sioux Center, Iowa. His speech was based on the epistle of Philemon, about the runaway slave Onesimus, and about how even the useless Onesimus became **useful** for the kingdom of God. Aly and I talked to Rev. Haan about our plans. I don't recall ever having received such positive encouragement regarding any of my plans, not before or afterwards. Slowly my dream of becoming a teacher started to become real. I sent my Dutch high school records to Dordt College; I was accepted for the fall of 1961. But it wasn't until we sold the bakery that we moved to Sioux Center, Iowa. It was August of 1962, and I was

30 years old.

In 1966 after graduation with a Bachelor of Arts in Education we moved to Lynden, Washington, where I taught German, math, and Bible at Lynden Christian High School. I then earned a Master's degree in German at the University of Washington, and in the fall of 1969 Dordt College hired me to teach German and eventually Dutch. I earned another Master's degree in 1975, this one in linguistics from the University of North Dakota. I obtained my Doctor of Arts at the State University of New York in Applied Linguistics while on sabbatical from 1982–3. The last fifteen years at Dordt I supervised the SPICE program, a semester offered in the Netherlands focusing on European language, history, and culture. We coordinated the students' excursions into the Dutch environment and provided care and management of the program and the students as well. I retired from teaching in 2000 and moved to Vernon, British Columbia in 2002. We were happy to be nearer our family.

Throughout my life as baker and professor, as father and husband, I have sought to serve the Lord. After I was diagnosed with Parkinson's disease, I felt that even in this situation I could be **useful** to others. My intent with this book is to help others by sharing the story of God's faithfulness to me, to provide information about Parkinson's and how to live with it positively, and to encourage family and friends and those who have Parkinson's disease. This book is my way of responding to the Lord's call to serve Him and others. Please join me now as we begin "sharing the road" in a journey through Parkinson's disease.

Case J. Boot
March 2011

CHAPTER 1
THE JOURNEY BEGINS:
TEACHING WITH HURDLES

This story tells about a physical disorder that invaded my life and sent me on an unexpected detour in my journey. To me it seemed that some strange power had commandeered parts of my rather wholesome body and steered it off the course I intended. I was determined to remain positive throughout these unusual encounters. I recognized that, no matter what may come, I had to choose a way to respond to these events. Initially I was quite sure that I should not bother my wife, Aly, with these experiences. I hoped that I might be in for some intriguing surprises, since up to this point my life had been blessed with many interesting events. As I write this account today, I am still unsure which approach I should have taken. This book is the story of my ongoing journey with Parkinson's disease, and it's my way of sharing some "travel tips" with the readers of this story.

The first time that I felt I was not in control of my fine motor skills was in an early morning linguistics class during the fall semester of 1996. I was in my twenty-seventh year of teaching at Dordt College, a small liberal arts college in Sioux Center, Iowa. Like the students, I too was fighting off yawning. I was explaining the assigned exercises when a student interrupted and spoke up rather loudly from the back of the classroom. "Sir," he asked, "why are you writing so small?" I stopped, took a few steps back and examined my writing. The student was correct. From then on I paid closer attention to the size of my writing, being sure to make it clear and large enough for students to read information from the blackboard.

My hand felt forced to write small on paper as well. Especially consistent was my struggle in writing with a felt pen on transparencies for the overhead projector. The pen skidded on the slippery surface. It was as if some mischievous power was interfering with my motor skills. In my mind I cursed this imaginary pest that was playing games with me. I wondered if it was going to be necessary to engage in open warfare, or whether I should stay in the trenches and prepare for a surprise attack from this unknown enemy!

Somehow I struggled through the remainder of the semester. Writing more slowly would help me to write larger, but this would cost important classroom minutes. Every class period has fifty minutes, even for teachers who have skirmishes with imaginary writing pests. I began to write fewer notes on quizzes and tests and would instead make oral comments to the whole class.

Up until this time in my career, I had been proud of my clear writing skills on any medium. Now I faced feelings of failure. It seemed I must be prepared for surprises. Was this something temporary? While wishing that the semester would end soon, I decided not to despair but to anticipate happier days ahead.

Although I was looking forward to a new beginning, the second semester would be challenging. I was once again in charge of Dordt's semester abroad program in Europe—Study Program in Contemporary Europe (SPICE)—with an enrollment of twenty-five students from a variety of colleges and universities. We would be living in Amsterdam in the Netherlands. My responsibilities included scheduling classroom time at the Free University and coordinating excursions for the art, architecture, history, culture, and business courses. Also, I taught Dutch language courses. My wife Aly and I were in charge of student housing and also hosting the SPICE office in our apartment. Administering SPICE meant adjusting to the Dutch bureaucratic system; to add to the confusion, many rules kept changing from year to year and only a few administrators would explain the new rules.

It was January. As I prepared for the Dutch language courses, I was relieved that most work was oral, and I was determined to use the blackboard sparingly. Transparencies were prepared the evening before, and I managed to muddle through. I had not yet shared my writing problem with anyone, not even with Aly.

Near the end of the semester I went to the bank to take care of some routine business. The clerk asked me to sign a few forms. A shaky, micrographic copy of my signature was the result. I did my best to make my signatures look genuine, but it was no longer what it once was. Why didn't my signature flow out of my pen automatically like it always had? Fortunately, the clerk recognized me. I told him that I had cold hands. "Yes, indeed, it is that time of year," he responded. I was concerned that the smooth, flowing signature I had developed since my high school days was forever gone. Back then, in my optimistic way, I had imagined that this signature would someday authorize banks to make large financial transactions. *Yes, I've always been a dreamer.*

On my way home, I thought about the signing incident. It felt like the same little pest was steering my signing hand astray, much like my miniature writing on the blackboard. But, there was no pain in my hand.

I was home in time to catch the five o'clock news. There was a health report on movement disorders, and it included a recent medical report on Prince Claus, husband of Queen Beatrix, who had been diagnosed with Parkinson's disease a few years earlier. All I knew about Parkinson's was that most patients had a tremor or a slight shake in one of their hands. According to the report, Prince Claus had several visible symptoms that were typical of Parkinson's patients; it was predicted that his condition would gradually deteriorate.

According to the report, Parkinson's disease patients may

have "facial masking"; they would not smile as readily as previously. I immediately checked my face in the mirror. Did I have the Pepsodent smile? Or, did I look like a grumpy humbug? I did not think so, nor did I think that I had a masked face. My students and I had many occasions to laugh; I felt I could pass this first test with flying colours.

Also, many Parkinson's disease patients would not swing their arms when walking. The hand from the non-swinging arm would be held close to the rigid body, and it would be shaped like a tent. The next morning on my walk to the University I decided to examine the swinging/non-swinging arm phenomenon. What a hopeless task! Some who walked near me had one hand holding their briefcase and the other hand in their coat pocket. Others had both hands in their pockets. Others would swing their free arm, I imagined, to the melody of "Oh, What a Beautiful Morning!" Indeed, it was a good morning, but the morning's observations did not provide satisfactory data for my research.

That evening, the 4th of May, I went to the Dam Square in Amsterdam, where I could observe Prince Claus. He would be accompanying the Queen at the wreath-laying ceremony at the National World War II Monument. Prince Claus took very small steps, as if he was rushing to get somewhere. His body looked rigid, and he had a slightly bent posture. His right shoulder bent forward, and his face was masked.

I was reasonably sure that my posture was closer to normal than Prince Claus's, but how much longer would it be so? Even now, when my hand was at rest, my pinky finger would tremble slightly. Would this tremor soon become more like a shake? Often, my writing was smaller; my arms no longer swung satisfactorily. According to the news report, I would "lose ground."

Parkinson's disease affects a person's emotional expression. One evening I went for a walk. I paused to watch a duck with her ten ducklings; I stood there, admiring God's creation while tears rolled down my cheeks.

During this time, my mind teeter-tottered between hopefulness and desperation. I wondered if living with Parkinson's would still provide me with opportunities for service, somehow, somewhere. I became convinced that teaching with a handicap like Parkinson's could be acceptable and serviceable in education. Then, one night, a nightmare forced me to face my fears. In my dream I saw that *The Banner*, the monthly magazine for my church denomination, displayed a quarter page ad for my teaching position. I, myself, had created a vacancy for my own position.

Once the semester was completed, we made preparations to leave Amsterdam. Aly is a very well-organized housekeeper, and when she is packing she would rather have her husband mind his own affairs. Although there was much to do, it was my pattern to take time off to help myself prepare for the return to North America. I would spend time at the Rijksmuseum to appreciate once more the works of seventeenth-century Dutch artists. I would allow Rembrandt's "hidden light source" of *The Night Watch* to penetrate my tired mind. Visiting museums without a class of students provided opportunity for the paintings to leave deep impressions. This time, as I was experiencing unease about my symptoms, I knew that my thoughts would often return to these Dutch painters and to their works of art.

CHAPTER 2
WHAT IS THE DIAGNOSIS?

Upon returning home to Sioux Center, I wanted to find out more about my handwriting problem. My thumb and index finger would tremble slightly when turning a page in a book. Perhaps there would be a connection between that and my writing experiences.

I had also promised my wife that I would make an appointment with our family doctor. Both Aly and a good friend from the SPICE program in Amsterdam, Aukje Bos, had been saying that I looked exhausted. I always put a lot of stock in advice from women, especially when Aly and Aukje were in agreement. Because of the clinic's vacation schedule, we would need to wait a few weeks for an appointment, which suited me fine. We made plans to travel to Red Deer, Alberta.

Staying with Harry and Willie at their hobby farm in Red Deer had always been a special treat for Aly and me, especially after our busy semester in Amsterdam. Spending time with the farm animals was a good way for me to slow down. It also gave me an opportunity to reflect and wonder why my body behaved the way it did.

That summer Harry and Willie celebrated their 35th wedding anniversary. For the occasion, I was the designated anniversary cake decorator. I had learned this craft while working in bakeries shortly after my immigration to Canada. The ladies of the house gave me the whole kitchen and provided all the necessary ingredients; they had gone shopping, so they would not be looking over my shoulder (which can be very annoying and distracting).

Soon I discovered that I was having difficulty holding the

decorating tool. Cake decorators must use both hands in a co-ordinated way, but I was no longer able to make a straight line or write "Happy Anniversary" to my satisfaction. After several attempts I gave up and decided it would have to be good enough. Willie and Aly commended my efforts, but it did not pass my standards. Was there a connection between writing with chalk on the blackboard, writing with pen or pencil on paper, and decorating a cake? I felt as if I was failing in all of those motor skills.

Writing on the blackboard involves hand movement. Writing with pen or pencil on paper or felt pen on a transparency includes finger movement. Writing on a cake requires both hands. Definitely my hands were shaking much more during the cake-decorating incident than when writing on the blackboard or paper. My hands had been moving up and down violently while writing "Happy Anniversary" and making swirling designs. This was disappointing and shocking because my handwriting had not deteriorated during the past semester.

Once we were back in Iowa, I kept my appointment with our family doctor. I shared the information about feeling tired, but he must have suspected some neurological problems. He immediately made an appointment for me with a neurologist in Sioux Falls, South Dakota.

The following week the neurologist instructed me to walk up and down the hallway several times. He asked me to do what I would call finger gymnastics. I had to point at my nose several times from various angles. I was not the least bit worried about missing my nose because mine is a size large. The nurse recorded a lot of data on her clipboard and, after a twenty-minute wait (supposedly to make the verdict sound authoritative I thought), the neurologist informed me that I had been diagnosed with Parkinson's disease. In a very offhand manner he handed me my first prescription. I felt as if he was awarding me a diploma of excellence of some sort.

The neurologist wondered why I was not surprised or

shocked by this diagnosis. I told him about my handwriting experiences, but I did not tell him what I had learned about Prince Claus. He did not strike me as one who would be interested in stories about the European monarchs.

Since that first morning when my blackboard writing was "off," I had been listening to stories about Prince Claus and others affected by Parkinson's disease. Although I had not opened a book on the topic, I was aware that from now on I could expect changes. The diagnosis did not really upset Aly, either. She too had suspected that my symptoms might be evidence of Parkinson's disease.

Life together would be taking a different direction, not one that we had been anticipating. We calmly agreed that Parkinson's disease is not a death sentence but an invitation and a challenge to a new and unfamiliar lifestyle. Even so, on the way home from Sioux Falls, I choked up. I raised my fist to God and cried out to Him, "How can you do this, Lord?" This reaction, too, was part of the journey we traveled.

We decided to gather more firsthand information on what it was like to live with Parkinson's disease. In northwest Iowa we knew of several gentlemen living with this condition. So, Aly and I made arrangements to visit with them.

Our first visit was with Henry, a man about my own age. He had worked as a clerk for an agency before his retirement; he had a wide spectrum of interests. He loved watching birds in his backyard and appreciated visitors, especially those with good stories to tell. Henry's hands would quiver slightly, and he had a drooling problem. Recently, it had become difficult for him to swallow his food. Aly and I imagined that Henry's case was quite normal for a late onset of Parkinson's. Henry had consulted a neurologist who had prescribed appropriate medication.

We visited George as well. He had been a carpenter for many years. His Parkinson's symptoms were quite clear. He had shaking hands, jerky arm and leg movements, and speech difficulty. George did not seem to be busy with hobbies that he could still manage. George's family doctor had not urged him to meet with a neurologist, and he was taking only one Sinemet pill per day. I was reluctant to ask whether that was what the doctor had prescribed or if he was taking such a small dose because of the high cost of medication.

We also heard of someone who screamed very loudly and flailed his arms violently. Later we learned this behaviour was not uncommon. This frightened Aly.

Although our visits with these men were not encouraging, our time with Henry more closely matched the Parkinson's literature we had read. These men had adjusted with the help of their spouse, children, and friends. Whatever the degree of the symptoms, all Parkinson's patients needed strong social support.

After about a year of wondering whether or not my symptoms were indicators of Parkinson's disease, we now had a firm diagnosis. Aly and I were ready to make adjustments in our lifestyle as required. We would take one day at a time, knowing that the Lord is always with us.

I was able to continue with my work at Dordt College for several more semesters. The medication regime was successfully keeping the symptoms at bay. Determined physical activity such as regular walking and running was also effective therapy.

The people of our community were very curious about Parkinson's disease. I met others with the disease, and our conversations often included questions about diagnosis dates and a comparison of limitations brought on by the disease.

Eventually a replacement for my position at the college was found. By God's grace, I had been able to continue working until I was almost seventy years old.

In 2002, five years after the Parkinson's disease diagnosis, Aly and I made a decision to move to Vernon, British Columbia. It was a location that gave us easier access to family. We both had brothers and sisters and friends living in British Columbia and in Alberta. Our four children who are scattered across North America enjoyed coming to the beautiful Okanagan to spend time with us. Although Parkinson's disease has taken us into unknown and challenging territory, we remain determined to enjoy our retirement years.

We had to face new difficulties. During the summer of 2009, both Aly and I spent time in the hospital and underwent major surgery. Although our faith was tested, we had many surprises. We received support from friends, relatives, and people from our church. We were grateful for the healing process and experienced God's goodness every day. We found another road sign pointing us *homeward*. This time, we wondered if the sign pointed to our eternal home.

CHAPTER 3
WHAT ARE THE SYMPTOMS?

Upon my diagnosis, my natural curiosity led me to search for information about where I was heading in my Parkinson's journey. Besides visiting people I began to read up on the history and symptoms of Parkinson's disease.

In 1817 James Parkinson wrote, "Essay on the Shaking Palsy." He concentrated on the tremor: "He saw that with his patients this tremor would start with coming and going intervals, a trembling of one limb, and this tremor would eventually become uncontrollable."[11]

The symptoms vary widely from one patient to the next. Further research has shown that neurons are destroyed in a portion of the midbrain called the *substantia nigra* (black substance). Parkinson's disease comes from a disorder in this black substance. The large pigmented neurons undergo a mysterious degeneration, depriving the brain of a chemical called dopamine, which is produced in the black brain and is crucial to proper human movement.

The following are considered primary symptoms of Parkinson's disease:
- rigidity (stiffness)
- tremor (hands and feet, head, neck, face, lips, tongue, jaw)
- *bradykinesia* (slowness of movements)
- loss of balance

---

1 Abraham N. Lieberman and Frank L. Williams, *Parkinson's Disease: The complete guide for patients and caregivers* (New York: Philip Lief, 1993), p. 26. See also A. N. Lieberman, *Shaking up Parkinson's Disease: Fighting like a tiger, thinking like a fox* (Boston: Jones and Bartlett, 2001).

- loss of automaticity (the ability to move automatically without having to think about it).

The following are considered secondary symptoms:
- gait disturbances
- facial mask (lack of a spontaneous smile)
- dexterity and coordination difficulties
- freezing
- speech and swallowing dysfunction
- depression
- urinating difficulties
- constipation[2]

When possible, I will draw from my own experiences as I describe these primary and secondary symptoms.

Rigidity

Parkinson's patients often appear to be holding their body rather stiffly. The rigidity can affect all the smaller muscles of the body. The most obvious examples are the restricted movement of the arms when a patient is walking. Each time I visit the neurologist I am asked to walk up and down the hallway. I know that I should swing my arms when I walk. The specialist is quite aware of my efforts at faking swinging arms. Lately, my body is very rigid. This makes walking or moving from one sitting position to another difficult. Getting out of bed is also burdensome.

Tremor

The resting tremor may involve not only the head, voice, legs, and trunk but also the neck, face, lips, tongue, and jaw. The Essential Tremor (also known as the Familial Tremor) may be mistaken for the Parkinson's Tremor. It is common among seniors. But, it begins in the second, third, fourth, or fifth finger, whereas the Parkinson's Tremor begins in the thumb fol-

---

2   Ibid., p. 13

lowed by the pinky.[3] My first encounter with the tremor was turning the pages of a book. My thumb's slight tremor made it difficult to separate two pages.

Bradykinesia

This slowing of movement affects walking, speaking, sitting down, writing, and even speech. It takes much effort to make myself understood, and I have to concentrate on finishing the word, especially if it concludes with consonants. My writing has gradually deteriorated since my linguistics class and my signature attempts at the bank in Amsterdam. Now I wish for those days when my writing was micrographic but legible. Lieberman and Williams state that *bradykinesia* may even affect thought.[4]

Loss of Balance, Falling

While walking or standing, Parkinson's patients look for supports to lean on. It is difficult to stop a fall. I myself have experienced four serious falls. In each case, I fell forward and experienced injuries, some of which required hospitalization.

Loss of Automaticity

When walking from one point to another, people will automatically have an internal estimate about the distance to be covered and an opinion on the quality of the terrain. Parkinson's patients need to consciously calculate how many steps will be required to reach the destination. They will also need to evaluate if the surface is rough or smooth. The Parkinson's patient needs to think about efforts that were previously automatic. They need to reconsider how to walk and to take taller, longer steps; they may even need to count the steps as they proceed.

---

3   Ibid., pp. 13 & 14
4   Ibid., p. 15

Freezing (feature of Bradykinesia)

Parkinson's patients may experience unexpected, involuntary arrest of what is usually voluntary movement. They may freeze in their tracks and may then struggle to initiate or continue movement. This difficulty may range from movements as minor as finger tapping to speaking or walking through a doorway or navigating a sudden turn. The patients may also feel stuck to the floor when passing by a wall of tall furniture or when surrounded by a crowd of people. Once frozen, I attempt to take a step backwards by shifting my weight to the other foot and then counting 1, 2, 3, 4, as I begin walking forward again.[5]

Gait Disturbance

Many Parkinson's patients develop a slightly bent forward posture, especially while walking. This syndrome, considered to be one of the most disabling, is called festination. Patients seem to be walking "in a hurry" against their will. They may also shuffle their feet, which combined with their festination can result in a dangerous fall.[6]

Dexterity and Coordination Difficulties

Although this phenomenon is not a result of clumsiness, it does result in awkwardness when opening or closing buttons. I find that dressing at a mirror can somewhat alleviate the difficulties.[7]

Speech and Swallowing Dysfunction

Even in early stage Parkinson's disease, speech abnormalities may become noticeable. Muscles from the diaphragm to the oral and nasal cavity are involved with speech production. Whispering and slurred speech are common; speech may sound nasally due to the improper closure of the nasal cavity. The

---

5   Ibid., pp. 16 & 17.
6   Idem.
7   Ibid., p. 16.

speech may also lack expression and sound monotone. Muscles involved with speech are also used in swallowing. Because of the swallowing dysfunction, management of saliva is compromised. To help alleviate this problem, chewing gum and sucking on hard candy are recommended.[8]

Early symptoms can be controlled with medication. Some of the standard medication that might be the most suitable for patients who have been diagnosed earlier in their condition may cause different reactions in patients who have later symptoms.

Once you have been diagnosed with Parkinson's disease, it is critical to have a support network ranging from friends to disease experts. A list of such supporters could include a neurologist, your family doctor, a social worker, a clergyman, your spouse, a sibling, a colleague, a physiotherapist, the pharmacist, and a friend. Every day presents new challenges, but remaining as active as possible in one's profession and hobbies can help fend off discouragement.

The Parkinson's disease patient's support network may recognize and understand the symptoms more clearly by reading this letter:

Letter to My Friends,

I have Parkinson's disease. It is neither catching nor hereditary. No one knows what causes it, but some of the dopamine cells in the brain begin to die at an accelerated rate. Everyone slowly loses some dopamine cells as they grow older. If the cells suddenly begin to die at a faster rate, Parkinson's disease develops. It is slowly progressive and usually occurs as people get older. Medicine can help. I'll take newer, stronger kinds over the years. Some make me sick and take lots of adjustments. Stick with me. I have good days and bad days.

TREMORS : You are expecting me to shake. Maybe I will, maybe I won't. Medicine today takes care of some of the tremors. If

---

8   Ibid., p. 17.

my hands, feet, or head are shaky, ignore it. I'll sit on my hand or put it in my pocket. Treat me as you always have. What is a little shakiness between friends?

MY FACE : You think you don't entertain me anymore because I'm not grinning or laughing. If I appear to stare at you, or have a wooden expression, that's the Parkinson's. I hear you. I have the same intelligence. It just isn't as easy to show facial expressions. If swallowing is a problem, I may drool. This bothers me, so we'll mop up.

STIFFNESS : We are ready to go somewhere and, as I get up, I can hardly move. Maybe my medicine is wearing off; this stiffness or rigidity is part of the Parkinson's. Let me take my time. Keep talking. I'll get there eventually. Trying to hurry me won't help. I can't hurry. I must take my time. If I seem jerky when I start out, that's normal. It will lessen as I get moving.

EXERCISE : I need to walk every day. Walking two or three miles is good. Walk with me. Company makes walking fun. It may be a slow walk, but I'll get there. Remind me if I slump or stoop because I don't always know I'm doing it. My stretching, bending, pushing exercises must be done every day. Help with them if you can.

MY VOICE : As my deeper tones disappear, you'll notice my voice is getting higher and wispy. That's the Parkinson's. Listen to me. I know you can talk louder, faster, and finish my sentences for me. I hate that! Let me talk, get my thoughts together, and speak for myself. I'm still there. My mind is OK. Because I'm slower in movement, I talk more slowly too. I want to be part of the conversation. Let me speak.

SLEEPLESSNESS : I may complain that I can't sleep. If I wander around in the middle of the night, that's the Parkinson's. It has nothing to do with what I ate or how early I went to bed. I may nap during the day. Let me sleep when I can. I can't always control when I'm tired or feel like sleeping.

EMOTIONS : Sometimes I cry and appear to be upset, and you think you have done something to hurt my feelings. Probably not. It is the Parkinson's. Keep talking to me. Ignore the tears. I'll be OK in a few minutes.

Patience, my friend. I need you. I'm the same person; I've just slowed down. It's not easy to talk about Parkinson's, but I'll try if you want me to. I need my friends. I want to continue to be part of life. Please remain my friend.[9]

There is one friend who will never let you down. Day after day I receive my strength to go on from God, the God described in Psalm 23. He is the foundation of my support team. Leslie F. Brandt has written this contemporary version:

The Lord is my constant companion.
There is no need that he cannot fulfill.
Whether His course for me points
    to the mountaintops of glorious ecstasy
    or to the valleys of human suffering,
    he is by my side,
    he is ever present with me.
He is close beside me
    when I tread the dark streets of danger,
    and even when I flirt with death itself,
    he will not leave me.
When the pain is severe,
    he is near to comfort.
When the burden is heavy,
    he is there to lean upon.
When depression darkens my soul,
    he touches me with eternal joy.
When I feel empty and alone,
    he fills the aching vacuum with his power.
My security is in his promise
to be near me always,
and in the knowledge
that he will never let me go.[10]

9   Jean Wilkin, Parkinson Society of Southern Alberta, reprinted in newsletter from Southern Arizona Chapter of APDA.
10 Leslie F. Brandt, *Book of Christian Prayer* (Minneapolis: Augsburg, 1980), p.156.

Chapter 4
Medication Therapy

In September 1997, during my first class sessions of the semester, I made an announcement to the students concerning my physical situation. Although I felt as if I was making a confession, I simply said, "I have been diagnosed with Parkinson's disease. It is at the beginning stage, and I hope that the disease will not progress too quickly during this semester." For some students I may as well have said, "I am a Democrat," because that would have been more shocking for students from a predominantly Republican area of the American Midwest. At least I knew that the students were aware of the meaning of the word "Democrat," but they had no idea what "Parkinson's disease" meant. When asked, they associated it with people who have shaking hands.

When I was ready to leave the classroom, one of the students approached me. She said, "Mr. Boot, my grandpa also has Parkinson's. He does reasonably well, but it is not always easy for my grandma. I will be praying for you and your wife."

After thanking her, I suggested that we should talk sometime. For now, this made my day. At least there was one student who had some understanding of Parkinson's. I was grateful that she would be one of my prayer warriors for this semester.

In the summer of 1997, I had bought my first prescription to treat Parkinson's disease. It was a small dose of Sinemet 25/250 and I was to take it three times per day. Until now I had been experiencing very few troublesome physical symptoms of the disease. I did have a slight problem turning the pages of a book, but I felt fortunate that I didn't have visible tremors like a shaking hand. Because of the medication my writing had improved; no longer would students need to remind me to write larger. They did not notice that, at times, my thumb and index finger would not cooperate turning a page in my textbook. A colleague suggested that I should add "post-it" notes in my textbook. I also slowed down my writing, which helped me to write more clearly. My friends thought that I was very fortunate, and I agreed.

Neurologists usually begin prescribing a common starting dosage of Sinemet 25/100 two to three times daily to young patients who have shown symptoms of Parkinson's. Sinemet is a drug made up of two medications. The top (left) number of 25/250 indicates Carbidopa, and the bottom (right) number Levodopa. In this case, the patient receives 25 mg Carbidopa three times per day, and 250 mg Levodopa also three times per day. It is recommended that the Parkinson's patient take the medication one hour before mealtime with a glass of water. If the patient has gastro-intestinal distress, it is recommended that the medication be taken at mealtime.

The side effects could be periods of nausea, daytime sleepiness, involuntary movements, decreased appetite, and cramping. Some patients might experience hallucinations, confusion, and what they call the "on-off" effect.[1]

This is how the drug therapy works:

> The simplest and most direct way of treating the loss of dopamine, once produced within the *substantia nigra* cells, is to replace it with dopamine from another source. The drug Levodopa is converted in the brain to dopamine, replacing the dopamine once produced within the *substantia nigra*. *Levodopa* is now given in combination with *Carbidopa*, a substance that blocks the conversion of Levodopa outside the brain. This drug combination is called Sinemet. Today, virtually all patients with Parkinson's disease will eventually take the drug Sinemet.[2]

Recently, younger patients may often start with one of the

---

1   Lieberman and Williams, p. 54.
2   Ibid., p. 52.

newer dopamine agonists; the agonists are chemicals that bind to a receptor of the cell and trigger a response by that cell mimicking the action of the naturally occurring substance.

Since 2002 I have been taking Sinemet CR, a controlled release form of Sinemet. The range of daily dosage is 75–200 mg Carbidopa; 200–1,000 mg Levodopa. The Sinemet CR may be especially useful in patients with "on-off" effects.[3]

Lieberman compared the "on-off" with a light switch. "On" indicates the Sinemet is active, and "off" when it is not. With some Parkinson's patients, a more continuous flow of dopamine to the brain is helpful. Sinemet plus Comtan will enhance the "on" period. Comtan is available in 200 mg tablets. With each dose of Sinemet, patients take one Comtan 200 mg. In the beginning, Parkinson's patients start with 200 mg Comtan with every other dose of Sinemet and gradually build up to one Comtan for every Sinemet. Parkinsons's patients can take up to eight Comtans per day.[4]

Lieberman, when explaining the benefit of Comtan, adds:

> There is agreement that patients should start with Comtan when on-off starts. By preventing the lows (low blood and, presumably low brain levels of levodopa) of Sinemet, Comtan plus Sinemet may not only reduce on-off, but delay the appearance of on-off effects.[55]

Since May, 2010, I am taking the following medication with satisfactory results:

6:00 am - One Apo-levocarb 100/25 mg (chew)
One Sinemet CR 200/50
One Comtan 200 mg

The dose is repeated at 10:00 am, 2:00 pm, 6:00 pm, and 10:00 pm.

Taking the prescribed medication on time every time is critical. Doing so is so important that the Parkinson's Society

---

3   Ibid., p. 54.
4   Ibid., p. 224–225.
5   Ibid., p. 226.

of British Columbia has prepared a brochure for Parkinson's patients to take to the hospital should they need to spend time there (see Appendix 3). The brochure is addressed to all nursing staff.[6]

During my recent hospital stay, I was pleased that the nurses in charge of the medication took that responsibility very seriously. As the general population becomes more informed on the complexities of this disease, nurses, volunteers, and caregivers will be equipped to provide better care for the Parkinson's patients.

---

6 "PD Medication: Timing is Everything," brochure from the Parkinson Society of BC.

CHAPTER 5
PHYSICAL THERAPY

Medication therapy is only part of Parkinson's disease treatment. Even from the very beginning, I found physical exercise helpful for managing my symptoms and raising my spirits.

When thinking of physical exercise, you might have in mind the weekly half marathon run by your athletic neighbor or the early morning basketball training of your granddaughter or the after school practices of the high school football team. Some of these physical exercises might overlap with the prescribed exercises for Parkinson's patients, but *physical therapy* for Parkinson's patients involves specific exercises that play a therapeutic role in the patient's well-being.

First, the physical therapist assesses the patient's needs. Then the therapist considers how these needs may be alleviated by therapy and to what extent the exercises will benefit the participant. It is important to note that Parkinson's patients have no control of automatic actions. Actions that were previously automatic now require physical exercises that help train your mind.[1]

Aerobic exercises, such as walking, benefit not only Parkinson's patients but heart patients and others. These exercises can be enjoyed by anyone who has a chronic illness. During one of my daily walks with our poodle Dusty, a friend from our Parkinson's support group invited me to join the Smart Heart walking group. This group of two dozen or more people meets three times per week to walk for an hour; they then participate

---

1   John Argue, *Parkinson's Disease and the Art of Moving* (Oakland, CA: New Harbinger, 2000), p. 16.

in half an hour of exercises conducted by a physiotherapist.

Afterwards a group gathers for coffee, qualifying the gathering as a social event as well. We always have a great time sharing interesting stories and old jokes. Seniors can be very humorous!

In Iowa, I attended weekly small-group speech therapy sessions that were also helpful. The muscles involved with speech production undergo the same attrition as other body muscles; they become rigid. This affects the whole speech pattern. Volume may be reduced to a whisper. People often ask me to repeat what I've said. This may seem acceptable, but after many repeat requests my listening audience has certainly diminished. They become uncomfortable with having to ask me to repeat over and over again. I believe people have an irresistible urge to communicate, and listeners should persist with patience. I use a small electronic device that indicates voice decibel levels to monitor my own voice volume. Appendix 2 includes vocal exercises that I recommend.

Here are some guidelines for physical therapy as indicated by John Argue in his book. I have found them beneficial:

- Come to an internal stop, collect your attention, and relax all excitement.
- Imagine the action you have to do; remember and invent the best way to do it.
- With complete and focused attention, perform whatever action you need to do.
- Do that action gracefully, meaning the easiest way possible that still gets the job done.
- Complete the action and know when it is completed.
- Come to an internal stop and focus on the next action.[2]

Furthermore, Argue suggests that persons who get the job done with the least amount of fuss or force are performing *gracefully.*

---

2   Ibid., p. 16

Practical skills you will develop through Argue's program are:

- Taking natural, abdominal, full-blown breaths.
- Reaching steadily for success.
- Finding the easiest and safest way to perform an action.
- Being able to reverse direction at any moment.[3]

It is recommended that Parkinson's patients begin exercising as soon as they have been diagnosed. There are many Parkinson's disease exercise programs. John Argue's book has an excellent curriculum for these exercises. At the beginning of a new exercise, it might be more advantageous to have a friend or caregiver lead you through the exercise. In many communities there are programs available for a small fee. Commitment is important. Parkinson's patients must be committed to doing the exercises, and they must be committed to continue walking, biking, swimming, or performing another means of exercise.

Parkinson's patients wonder how these exercises are beneficial to them. John Argue gives a good answer to this question: *"It will help you anticipate, prevent, and delay symptoms."*[4] Argue stresses that the exercises prepare the patient physically to cope with the symptoms before they have arrived, or they may even prevent the emergence of the symptoms completely. An exercise program may reduce the harm done by certain symptoms and thus enhance a higher quality of life. Newly diagnosed persons are able to prepare themselves before the symptoms appear.

Parkinson's disease symptoms do not appear in tidy little packages. Every patient's experience and expression of symptoms is different. Some need exercises for the left pinky finger tremor, others for their left arm's swing, and yet others for the right hand's shaking. Patients may have to accept multiple health problems at various stages of their life. For example, arthritis in the right arm can prevent it from swinging. We need

---

3   Ibid., p. 17
4   Ibid., p. 19

to have a mental plan for our next move.

A look at daily traffic patterns can help describe a Parkinson's patient's situation. As a road narrows, traffic can become heavier and more challenging. We are fortunate here that a new road sign has been designed to deal with this situation. The traffic sign simply says: *SHARE THE ROAD*. It has symbols for a car and a bicycle. The sign is placed on the side of a road made up of one lane for cars in both directions, and one lane for bicycles in both directions, and a sidewalk for pedestrians.

When the road narrows there is only one lane in each direction for cars, no bicycle lane, and a narrow sidewalk for pedestrians on one side. Without interrupting the traffic flow, the people involved consider what their options are. There are some basic commonsense traffic rules that must be adhered to. This makes sense to those who use a car, a bike, or a pair of shoes in everyday traffic. It is very clear to them how to share the road. Those who are asked to share the road know instantaneously what their choices are and how to execute that choice. Parkinson's patients are confronted with similar challenges in their everyday movement.

What kind of obstacles do I encounter going from A to B? Two obstacles come to mind: my right leg freezes, and my left knee is the arthritic one, causing me pain. I suppose that the described obstacle prevents me from going ahead. No, not really! I simply shift my weight from the right of my body to my left, start an easy cadence, like 1, 2, 3, go, 1, 2, 3, go, 1, 2, 3, go, and rock myself out of this frozen state. I keep my toes pointing up and keep pushing toward the intended goal always with heel first and toe next. We need to have a mental plan.

The Parkinson's patient is not able to judge the distance automatically like she did before Parkinson became a reality in her life. My destination is about forty-eight steps away, and I continue counting following the cadence pattern: 1, 2, 3, go, 1, 2, 3, go, 1, 2, 3, go. I want to make sure that I have estimated the distance to point B quite closely. It has been suggested by some that you must select a point a short distance beyond point B; when you come to point B, you will realize you have achieved your intended target. You may congratulate yourself with this achievement.

At my first regional meeting of the Parkinson Society in British Columbia, there was an elderly person who seemed to be glued to the floor. He rocked his body back and forth, but he was unable to make the first step. I looked at him with pity; then I noticed that one of the speakers on the panel stuck out his foot. I was afraid – what was going to happen next, a football tackle? – but, to my surprise, the elderly person took a firm step forward; he was walking straight ahead to his target position. It was a normal walk. What made him take that first step, I asked myself. *The brain can do unimaginable things!*

You simply have to claim your share of the road. One of the ways you can do this is by stating out loud that you want to move from A to B. Or, you may address both your arthritic and Parkinson's opponents: "I am going to beat both of you next."

One needs to develop a strategy for dressing. Doing up buttons can be very challenging. I have learned to line up a button with the buttonhole, while keeping an eye on the mirror. Simply saying, "Sorry Bud, I've got to have this button, and that one, and a few more," might not do it for you. Somehow you have to keep this button-warfare at a fair game level. Velcro closings are also a practical solution. It is fine if Parkinson comes out on top once in a while, but in your mind you tell yourself that you are the next winner. It is all part of a fair game strategy.

Knotting a tie can also be a challenge, and it is one shared by many men. Although I must admit that I have never been committed to wearing a tie on a regular basis, there were occasions when wearing a tie was mandatory. I have become somewhat satisfied with my tie-tying abilities, and when I take my tie off, I simply pull my head through the big loop and hang the tie, still neatly tied, in my closet. Of course, the simplest route would have been not to be bothered with dressing up for special occasions. But, having Parkinson's does not mean that you have to cramp your style. We have to be determined to face obstacles along the way and to plan a strategy to deal with them. We can enjoy our life to the fullest. A properly tied tie might add flair to the occasion. I have a small collection of ties, and three of them are already tied, hanging in my closet. Always ready for a party!

Amid all the challenges and hard work and planning, I have found a huge advantage in having a positive attitude to life and realizing that Jesus is always present. When everything seems to be working against you, Jesus gives you strength for the day and hope for the future. The Dutch poet Geert Boogaard shares his view:

Suffering

There has never been
a training school
for suffering,
as if there is a God
who teaches you a lesson.
Hold on to a God
who has mercy
on you;
think about Jesus
who was sent by Him
and whom you could
find in your corner
where the hardest
blows struck.[5]

---

5   Geert Boogaard, *Niet zonder hoop* [Not Without Hope] (Nykerk: Callenbach, 1982), p. 53; translated from the Dutch.

CHAPTER 6
HOW, THEN, SHALL WE LIVE
WITH PARKINSON'S DISEASE?

We have seen that life with Parkinson's disease can disturb many aspects of ordinary life: it is a big change. It is up to the patient to find Parkinson's support groups. They need to find places to socialize and to exercise, places to share and to trade stories about treatments, symptoms, and experiences.

In my circle of acquaintances afflicted with Parkinson's, the happiest are those who are involved with all kinds of activities such as crafts, sports, and writing. Remaining involved in various aspects of society contributes to a meaningful life. The drug therapy, physical therapy, and aspects of vocations and hobbies contribute to a wholesome network of many interlocking cultural activities that result in a mosaic of satisfaction and joy. The lives of Parkinson's patients, in spite of the physical limitations, do not have to be dull or joyless.

It is an advantage to share the burden of Parkinson's with a spouse or with close relatives and friends. The caregivers need to temper their care with *tough love*. Wise and loving caregivers are sensitive and encourage the patient to remain independent for as long as possible.

For those of you who are caregivers, this sharing of the road enriches both of our lives. From the first encounter we realize how each of us functions. Sharing can provide opportunities unknown until now.

Making adjustments in your life to make living with Parkinson's possible prompts you to consider life from a new perspective. Having faith and believing in miracles also helps.

The following story is taken from the Bible's New Testament.

> One day as Jesus was teaching, Pharisees and teachers of the law, who had come from every village of Galilee and from Judea and from Jerusalem, were sitting there. And the power of the Lord was present for him to heal the sick. Some men came carrying a paralytic on a mat and tried to take him into the house to lay him before Jesus. When they could not find a way to do this because of the crowd, they went up on the roof and lowered him on his mat through the tiles into the middle of the crowd, right in front of Jesus.
>
> When Jesus saw their faith, he said, "Friend your sins are forgiven."
>
> The Pharisees and the teachers of the law began thinking to themselves, "Who is this fellow who speaks blasphemy? Who can forgive sins but God alone?"
>
> Jesus knew what they were thinking and asked, "Why are you thinking these things in your heart? Which is easier: to say, 'Your sins are forgiven,' or to say, 'get up and walk'? But that you may know that the Son of Man has authority on earth to forgive sins . . ." He said to the paralyzed man, "I tell you, get up, take your mat and go home." Immediately he stood up in front of him, took what he had been lying on, and went home praising God. Everyone was amazed and gave praise to God. They were filled with awe and said, "We have seen remarkable things today."
>
> Luke 5:17-26 (NIV)

A modern rendition could be the following:

> Once there was a young man who was diagnosed with Parkinson's disease. He had an early onset of the disease that eventually rendered him incapable of carrying out tasks that he had been able to do before.
>
> One of his friends who visited him suggested that he should ask a neurologist for a drug prescription that would help him control his writing, which had become a collection of mini-

graphics and close to illegible.

A second friend visited the Parkinson's patient and suggested that he join a group of Parkinson's patients who are involved with physical therapy. These therapists would work on exercising his muscles, which would help him overcome "freezing."

A third friend suggested that he get involved with a group of craftsmen like woodcarvers. Parkinson patients should keep their hands busy. They would make beautiful wooden bowls, which they could sell at craft fairs.

The Parkinson's patient and his friends were aware that God didn't need the means suggested by them. God is able to heal without the use of drugs, without any physical therapy, and without the patient doing woodwork. We believe that God is a Sovereign God and that he is able to use any means for healing.

What's needed is faith. We need to believe that miracles can occur. Pray for your friends afflicted with Parkinson's. Believe that God the Creator is powerful and can perform miracles. Bible stories have taught me that the Jesus, the Great Healer, forgives sins and heals the sick.

This healing may come through prescribed medication and physical exercise. If we take the proper medication and practice the proper physical exercises faithfully, we may *anticipate*, *prevent*, and *delay* Parkinson symptoms.[1] We hope that future research on medication and physical therapy may eliminate Parkinson's symptoms.

Parkinson's is a disease that progressively becomes more debilitating. I experience good days when the symptoms are not aggressive. To me, those days are miracles.

My friends need to recognize the presence of the Parkinson's symptoms:

- My masked face is not an indicator of me being unfriendly or dull.
- The surprising sobbing or crying does not make me a

1   Argue, p. 19.

crybaby.

- I may fall asleep, even while you are telling an interesting story; it doesn't mean that your story is boring to me.
- My whispering voice does not mean that I don't want to communicate with those who are hard of hearing.
- If you and I go for a walk, I may not be able to keep up with you, but your slower pace will help me enjoy the walk.
- My slow thinking process makes it difficult for me to keep up with conversations, but don't assume that I am not with it.
- My acquaintances expect one of my hands to be vigorously shaking. They assume that all Parkinson's patients have shaking hands. I am surprising them, although I do have slight tremors that are hardly noticeable.
- You need to be patient with me or other Parkinson's patients. Every patient may express different symptoms, although they may overlap.

I am grateful for the many good days I enjoy. I have found it important to share with my friends that their concern makes living with Parkinson's disease more bearable. I have found that the caregiver, the neurologist, the family doctor, friends, and relatives can all share the road with me.

Indeed, sharing the road with Parkinson's patients can be most satisfying.

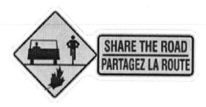

Sharing the Road

Sharing the road with each other,
takes only a little effort.
Each holds to the right,
and is concerned about safety
for those who walk or ride,
also for those who shuffle their feet.
I do recognize the humor in other voices
but I can't get a smile on my face.
All my deeper voices have disappeared,
you will notice that my pitch rises
and becomes whispery and dull.
Often I drool when I eat and
I feel the frowns directed at me,
but no one wipes my face.
I attempt to share a story,
but it takes others too long to listen.
Do my friends adjust to shuffling feet?
Keeping their same speed separates us,
slowing down builds community.
Handing someone a napkin to wipe
a drooling face, can be a basis of
understanding for a lifetime.
Laughing about it can lead to animosity.
There is development from little embraces,
to accepting one another as friends,
as creatures of one Creator and Lord.
This Creator does not control
Parkinson's from a distance.
This Creator is very close to you,
and strengthens you from day to day.

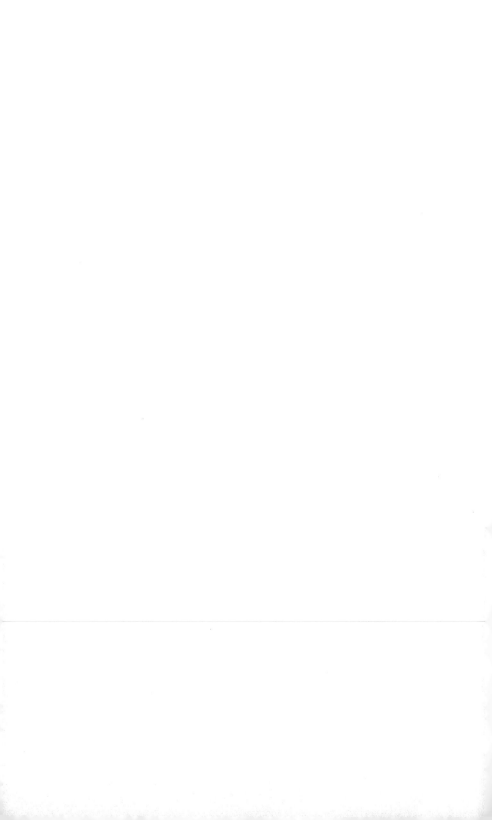

APPENDIX 1
MOVING FORWARD WITH PARKINSON'S – "PREVENTION TOWARDS PROGRESSION"[1]

A moving body will never stiffen...

Breathing

The muscles of the throat and chest usually have the same PD symptoms as the legs and hands—rigidity, slowness of movement, and incomplete range of motion (ROM).

For many people, their daily lives are filled with stressful situations, and whether they have PD or not, have learned to breathe shallow (known as the fight/flight response breathing) into their chest only.

The complete breath is a Yoga breathing exercise taught to enhance relaxation and to keep flexibility, strength, and suppleness to the spine and the muscles of respiration.

Belly Breathing

Sit tall and place your hands on your belly with fingers touching
  • Inhale slowly and push on your belly with fingers touching
  • Exhale slowly; pull belly button to spine
Repeat a few times.

Then place one hand on side of ribs. . .

This time as you breathe slowly, send your breath into your belly and then in to your rib cage. . . Repeat this a few times. Take hand from belly and place onto chest. . .

Continue breathing the same way but include the rise and fall of your chest as well. Notice the relaxation that comes from

---

1   Reproduced here with permission from Rhona Parsons CPT.

breathing this way.

The hand positions help you learn where to send your breath and to notice what your body is doing.

You may also notice that when you breathe in, your spine gently arches (this helps expand your rib cage) and when you breathe out, your belly pulls in towards your spine, using the abdominals to send your diaphragm up to send the breath out.

Foot/Ankle Exercises
Balance begins with our foundation—our feet. This first exercise is not only going to loosen your feet, but wake up the nerve endings for your whole body.

Ball under foot: done barefoot
This exercise is especially beneficial if you have poor circulation in your feet.
- Sit forward on the edge of your chair
- Place a tennis ball under the center of your foot
- Begin to roll the ball under your foot back and forth from heel to toes
- When you find a "hurt so good" spot, press down with your foot, leaning slightly forward to enhance the pressure
- Continue for 2–3 minutes

Notice how your ankles feel—not so tight and rigid?
- Take your foot off the ball and place it on the floor
- Feel the floor with your entire foot
- Repeat the exercise with your other foot

This exercise keeps your ankles flexible and strong.

Ankle Alphabet
- Sit tall but relaxed in your chair
- Keep leg straight and still and lift off the floor
- Draw the alphabet with your foot—the movement coming from your ankle; try to keep the leg still

Repeat with other leg.

Spine Stretches
- Sit tall in your chair, spine long
- Intertwine your fingers
- Exhale and straighten arms, pressing palms forward
  - A. Inhale and stretch up to the ceiling
  - B. Exhale, round your spine, and bring arms out to the front

Repeat A and B 3x, then:

- Inhale and stretch up to the ceiling
  - A. Exhale and bend to one side keeping your buttocks on the chair
  - B. As you inhale, feel your side expanding…
  - C. Exhale and bend to the other side
  - D. Inhale, expand your side
  - E. Exhale; come back to centre

Repeat 3x

Rotation
- Sit tall facing sideways in your chair, hands touching the back of the chair
- With each complete breath begin to twist your hips to the back of the chair, then your ribcage, then shoulders, and then head. . . . Inhale.
- Exhale and unwind your body. *Repeat 2x.*
- Repeat on other side

Arm Extensions
- Sitting tall with your hands on your shoulders, inhale and turn upper body and head to the right
- Exhale and reach your arm out straight behind you
- Inhale, hand back to shoulder
- Exhale and turn to centre

Repeat on left side. Repeat on both sides 3x

Leg Stretches
Hamstrings: sitting
- Sit tall in your chair
- Straighten out one leg; heel to floor, toes up
- Lean forward from your hips, keeping spine long and tall
- Push buttocks back and up
- Hold the stretch for 10–15 seconds
- Repeat on the other leg

Coming to Standing
- Sit at edge of chair
- Bring heels back so they're behind your knees
- Hands to thighs
- Lean forward, placing your weight in your hands and push up through your feet and hands to standing
- Keep your weight forward as you stand
- Stand up leaning forward and roll up spine

Feet rolling combo
- Stand behind chair, holding on with both hands
- Bend your knees
- Lift your heels
- Stand tall
- Place heels back on floor

Repeat 3x; then:
- Lift heels
- Bend knees
- Roll through feet to heels
- Stand tall

Calf stretches
- Stand behind chair, holding on with both hands
- Press right leg back as far as you can, pushing heel to floor
- Keep chest proud and lean forward
- Hold for 15–30 seconds
- Repeat with other leg

Appendix 2
Parkinson's Disease and Voice

Yawn
1. Make the full yawn "AHHHH" sound!

2. Spread open your hands as if you are holding a tennis ball:
   a. Notice that the stretching of your hands is similar to the stretching of your throat. Now stretch your hands and stretch your throat.
   b. The greatest similarity of stretching you will find in the midst of a good yawn
      Ahhh—AHHHH—Ahhhh

3. Larynx
   a. In the lowest position during a yawn
   b. In the highest position when you swallow

4. Benefits of yawning:
   a. Diaphragmatic breathing
   b. Speaking with full volume
   c. Improves swallowing
   d. Relaxing your muscles

5. Singing the AHHHH sound:
   a. Warm-up exercise making your own high-mid-low pitches
   b. Choose a song
      "London Bridge is falling down"
      "Jingle bells"
      "Oh what a beautiful morning"
      Add your songs

6. Practice these exercises at home!
   a. Sit forward on the edge of the chair
   b. Pretend you are making the AHHHH yawn without

the AHHHH sound

  c. Hold AHHHH on a singing pitch for about ten seconds

  d. Pretend you are a great opera singer and your voice goes up and down the ladder on AHHHH.

  e. Select from the following songs:
"I've been working on the Railroad"
"Old Macdonald had a farm"
"A Mighty Fortress is our God"
"Jingle Bells, Jingle Bells"
Others
Keep it going! Make it fun!

  f. Amazing Grace
Amazing grace, how sweet the sound
That saved a wretch like me!
I once was lost but now I'm found
Was blind but now I see.

  g. London Bridge
London Bridge is falling down,
Falling down, falling down
London Bridge is falling down.
My fair lady!

7. Test for volume!

  a. Sing three songs on a variety of AHHHH pitches.

  b. Try to speak the third song in a normal tone.

  c. Surprise: the volume increases

  d. Keep on practicing daily.

  e. Tired?
Probably a little sore in your ribcage or at your diaphragm!
It hurts so good.

Information based on Lesson 2, especially Ex. 2.2, pp. 70-71, *Parkinson's Disease and the Art of Moving,* by John Argue.

APPENDIX 3
PD MEDICATION: TIMING IS EVERYTHING

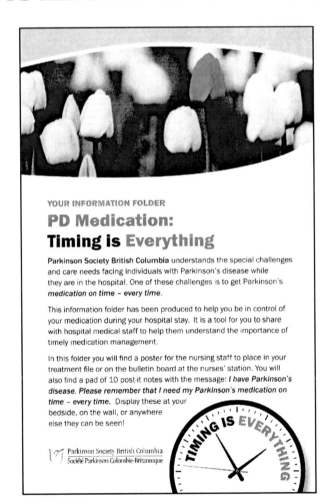

This page from the booklet "PD Medication: Timing is Everything" is reproduced with the written permission of Parkinson Society British Columbia (www.parkinson.bc.ca).

ACKNOWLEDGEMENTS

This sharing of my experiences regarding Parkinson's disease has taken on characteristics of a journey, too. There were travelers sharing the road with me, and I would like to acknowledge them:

- My certified personal trainer Rhona Parsons has provided much inspiration in regards to how effective the exercises are in anticipating, preventing, and delaying symptoms.
- Greg Johnson BSP, a local pharmacist, has kept me informed on and supplied me with the necessary medication therapy.
- Bob McDougall kept reminding me that a book such as this may give moral support to Pd patients.
- Andrew Vander Leek, pastor of East Hill Community Church, has provided a listening ear and much spiritual encouragement.
- My parents, who introduced me to the children's stories of the Bible, left their imprints on my life.
- Harry and Willie introduced us to a more relaxed lifestyle and to the joy of daily work.
- Linda Ensing, Clare Kooistra, and Linda Samland have helped me to polish my manuscript and helped prepare it for submission to the publishers.
- The enthusiasm of President B.J. Haan, President of Dordt College, who was a constant reminder to me to be positive in my studies and look out for impossible adventures in life.
- I want to express my sincere thanks to Corkie Huisman-Hentges, Dal Apol, and John Struyk—former

colleagues in the Foreign Language Department at Dordt College—for their strong opinions regarding the "nature of language." Some of their remarks seemed to come straight from Paradise. Without these discussions the departmental meetings would have been less interesting and much less educational.

- I want to acknowledge Paul Jones of the Vernon Parkinson Support Group who encouraged me with the writing of this book.
- I want to thank Aukje Bos-Geertsema for her enthusiasm in her art course and for her dedication to SPICE.

And through this entire journey and book process my dear wife Aly has been my number one medical caregiver and faithful supporter.